Radiant
Spirits
A Journey into Animal Reiki

ELIZABETH SELDEN

ISBN: 9798866749720
Independently Published

DEDICATION

For all the fuzzy, scaly, feathery beings I have had the honor of connecting with over the years and the human facilitators who brought us together. Sharing your space and energy is my honor and supporting you in restoring balance and harmony within your beings fills me with gratitude. Light, divinity, and healing are ours to share in these beautiful moments. May this text honor your grace.

CONTENTS

ACKNOWLEDGMENTS

Thank you to the many shelter pups and cats who nuzzled into my lap for a session after surgery, to the foster dogs who found love in our home for too short a time, to our "foster-fail" pup, and our ever-tolerant cats, my long-suffering husband, and children…who accepted it all…thank you.

Without exemplary training and years of professional experience across the United States and Japan, I would never have been able to master this powerful, beautiful, restorative, and ancient healing art. I am grateful for each experience and connection.

1 THE HISTORY OF REIKI

Reiki, pronounced "ray-key," is a holistic healing practice that originated in Japan in the early 20th century. The word "Reiki" is composed of two Japanese characters: "rei," which means universal or spiritual, and "ki," which means life force energy. Reiki, then, can be understood as "universal life force energy," representing the vital energy that flows through all living beings.

At its core, Reiki is based on the belief that this universal life force energy can be channeled and utilized for healing, relaxation, and overall well-being. It operates on the premise that disruptions or imbalances in the flow of this energy within the body can lead to physical, emotional, and spiritual ailments. Reiki aims to restore harmony and balance to these energy pathways, thereby promoting health and vitality.

While Reiki as a formalized practice emerged in the 20th century, the concept of manipulating and harnessing life force energy for healing has ancient roots. Various cultures throughout history have recognized the existence of a vital energy that animates all living things. In Chinese medicine, it is referred to as "Qi" or "Chi," in Ayurveda, it is known as "Prana," and in Greek philosophy, it was referred to as "pneuma."

These ancient healing traditions understood the importance of maintaining the balance and flow of this vital energy for optimal health. Practices such as acupuncture, qigong, and yoga all share the fundamental principle of working with this life force energy to promote well-being.

The specific practice known as Reiki, however, was developed by Mikao Usui, a Japanese Buddhist monk and spiritual seeker, in the early 20th century. Usui's journey toward discovering Reiki began with a profound spiritual experience on Mount Kurama in Kyoto, Japan.

Legend says that in the year 1922, after a 21-day meditation and fasting retreat on the mountain, Usui experienced a powerful enlightenment. During this transformative experience, he received the knowledge and ability to channel Reiki energy. This event marked the birth of the formalized Reiki system.

Usui's approach to Reiki emphasized not only the physical healing aspects but also the spiritual growth and self-realization that could be achieved through the practice. This holistic approach contributed to the enduring effectiveness of Reiki as a now widely accepted healing modality.

Studies have shown that Reiki sessions, lasting anywhere from 15 to 60 minutes, can lead to a reduction in heart rate, blood pressure, and levels of stress hormones like cortisol. This suggests that Reiki may activate the parasympathetic nervous system, promoting a state of deep relaxation and facilitating the body's natural healing processes.

Research participants have reported improvements in areas such as mood, sleep quality, emotional well-being, and overall vitality. These findings suggest that Reiki may offer holistic benefits that extend beyond the physical realm alone.

2 UNDERSTANDING ENERGY

There is often a misconception about the definition of "energy." The layman hears this term and disregards it as an intangible concept having little practical value or application.

Self-help gurus define "energy" as a certain quality of life or a measurement of action or a step-by-step process followed to change an individual's current life path trajectory.

Spiritualists understand "energy" to mean that all things in the universe carry a specific vibration through which they naturally interact because they are inherently connected.

The Metaphysician determines the value of energy existing in each of these forms and the nature of its impact on other forms. Because of the essence of our existence, all things constantly influence one another causing either harmony or separation.

Thoughts = Energy
Words = Energy
Emotions = Energy
Food = Energy
Action = Energy
The Elements (Earth, Water, Air, Fire & Spirit) = Energy
All Living Things = Energy
All Inanimate Objects = Energy

But how can this information be practically applied to healing, to Reiki itself?

The practitioner of Eastern medicine will tell you your body is made up of certain elements. Each element is comprised of very specific energies. If any one of those elements is out of balance, the physical body, mental body, emotional body, and eventually the spiritual body can become ill.

Reiki assists in rebalancing and restoring the energies that are out of alignment, creating an opportunity for deep healing to occur. A skilled practitioner can identify and isolate hotspots while also stimulating a deep, whole-being healing process.

Holistic therapies are a whole-person/whole-being approach to health, working together with diet, exercise, western medicine, and other holistic therapies to provide a tailored and effective experience for each individual.

Because everything we consume, think, and encounter impacts the nature and quality of our energy, the more present we are, the more aware we will be when our energy begins to change. In this state, we will be able to mediate adjustments before a negative shift impacts our health or well-being.

Concerning our animal companions, the same is true. Animals are experts at sharing their state of mind and body. We must simply pay attention to the signs they provide.

Some imbalances in animals can appear as follows:

- Anxiety: pacing or restlessness, excessive grooming, hiding, loss of appetite, agitation or aggression, excessive vocalization, toileting issues, destructive behavior, withdrawal, trembling, tense body language, elevated heart rate or respiration

- Depression: lack of interest in play, changes in sleeping patterns, decreased appetite, withdrawal or avoidance, excessive grooming, weight loss or gain, lethargy, destructive behavior, change in vocalizations, hiding, lack of response to stimuli, listlessness, social withdrawal

- Illness: loss of appetite, sudden weight loss, refusal to eat, vomiting, diarrhea, lethargy, weakness, changes in urination, coughing, sneezing, labored breathing, changes in grooming, aggression or withdrawal, changes in gait, expressing pain vocally, changes in feces, swelling, lumps

Reiki is Light. The practitioner moves into a meditative state through which s/he connects with and then channels the Reiki Ray through her/his own body and directs it into the client.

Modern Reiki practitioners may use a series of symbols, while those following the original practice of Mikao Usui, will use very few, if any.

Regardless of how the Reiki Ray is anchored and transmitted to the client, the important thing to understand is that the Light is anchored and then channeled into the client's energetic field, gently penetrating the physical and mental bodies as necessary.

The Light energy sustained through the practice of Reiki naturally restores balance. It creates harmony and allows healing to occur by resetting the frequencies of the body and mind.

Reiki provides a natural, sacred, non-invasive, and completely safe experience that can be incorporated seamlessly with any other healing modality for improved success and sometimes even miraculous results.

3 ANIMAL SPIRITS

Animals, like humans, are highly sensitive to energy. They exist in a state of natural attunement with the environment, making them receptive to the healing energies of Reiki. The practice of offering Reiki to animals recognizes and respects this innate sensitivity.

The heightened ability to perceive energy fields and vibrations allows animals to pick up on subtle shifts in their environment, the emotions of humans and other animals, and changes in their own bodies. Animal Reiki practitioners leverage this natural sensitivity to facilitate healing and promote well-being.

Animal Reiki offers a range of potential benefits for animals, including:

- Stress Reduction: Just like humans, animals can experience stress and anxiety. Reiki provides a calming and soothing energy that helps alleviate these feelings.
- Pain Management: Reiki can be effective in managing pain, whether it is due to injury, illness, or the aging process.
- Emotional Balancing: Animals, especially those with traumatic pasts, can experience emotional wounds. Reiki helps address these emotional imbalances and promotes a sense of security and trust.
- Enhanced Well-Being: Reiki supports overall physical and emotional well-being, helping animals lead happier and more fulfilling lives.

- Complementary to Veterinary Care: Reiki is often used as a complementary therapy alongside conventional veterinary treatments. It can enhance the effectiveness of medical interventions and speed up the healing process.

Practicing Reiki with animals requires a unique approach, as animals communicate, respond, and often receive energy differently than humans. As a practitioner, I take each of the following into consideration with each animal I serve, each time I am in service:

- Non-Invasive Approach: Reiki is non-invasive, meaning the practitioner does not need to touch the animal. This also makes it possible for me to perform this work very successfully on a remote basis as needed.
- Respect: Practitioners must observe the animal's body language and behavior to gauge their level of comfort. When an animal has received enough for the session, it is important to observe the signs being given and to end the energy flow at that time.
- Creating a Healing Space: A calm and peaceful environment is essential for successful Reiki sessions. Minimizing distractions and providing a comfortable space helps the animal feel at ease. It is always my preference to perform sessions in the client's home or familiar space whenever possible.

Animal Reiki can be applied to a wide range of animals, including domestic pets, farm animals, wildlife, and even marine life. Each species has unique needs and responses to the energy, but each can receive and respond to the natural patterns of attunement.

This practice is a testament to the universal applicability of a beautiful and ancient healing art. By extending the benefits of Reiki to animals, practitioners contribute to the harmony of all living beings on our planet.

4 THE ART OF COMMUNICATION

In the realm of understanding and connecting with animals, there exists a unique and profound form of communication known as animal communication. This practice transcends verbal language, allowing humans to tap into the unspoken thoughts, emotions, and sensations of our animal companions. By doing so, it offers a gateway to a deeper level of mutual understanding.

Animals communicate through a rich tapestry of non-verbal cues, body language, and energy exchanges. While humans have developed various methods to interpret these signals, the practitioner of animal communication takes this understanding to a different level. The skilled practitioner gains direct access to an animal's thoughts, feelings, and physical sensations, bridging the gap between our species.

At the heart of animal communication lies empathy—an ability to step into the paws, feathers, scales, or hooves of our animal friends. This practice encourages humans to set aside preconceived notions and truly listen, without the constraints of language as we define it. By doing so, we can gain a more profound understanding of an animal's experiences, desires, and needs.

One of the most valuable aspects of animal communication is its healing potential. Animals, like humans, carry emotional wounds, traumas, and anxieties. Through communication, practitioners can offer better support, reassurance, and a safer space for animals to express themselves and receive healing. This can lead to immediate and lasting shifts in behavior and deep positive changes in emotional well-being.

Many animals exhibit behavioral challenges that stem from past experiences, fears, or unmet needs. Animal communication can be an invaluable tool in unraveling the root causes of such behaviors. By addressing the underlying issues, humans can work together with their animal companions to find solutions that promote harmony and balance.

Most importantly, the practice of animal communication nurtures a deep and mutual bond between humans and their animal companions. It fosters a sense of trust, respect, and cooperation that goes beyond mere companionship. This heightened connection often leads to more fulfilling and enriched relationships between humans and their animal companions of any breed.

Animal Reiki often goes hand-in-hand with animal communication. Combining these modalities can lead to deeper insights and a more comprehensive approach to holistic animal care.

It is important to note that animal communication is not a one-sided endeavor. Animals are adept at communicating with humans through their own intuitive channels and do so with their every interaction. By honing our receptive abilities, we open ourselves to a dynamic exchange of thoughts, feelings, and energies, creating a true partnership for healing and so much more.

If you are interested in embarking on this transformative journey with your animal companion, simply follow the steps below to get started:

1. Choose a quiet, comfortable space free from distractions for both you and the animal. Be seated comfortably within a safe view and distance of the animal.
2. Quiet your mind and center your energy within your central core (the center of your body—all along your spine).
3. Take three deep, slow breaths in through your nose and release just as slowly through your mouth, closing your eyes and relaxing your body as you do so.
4. Let go of any thoughts passing through your mind at this time, simply breathing them through without judgment.
5. When you feel stillness within, acknowledge the animal sharing your space. The more centered you are and the more your energy is focused within your central core, the calmer the animal will also be. Acknowledgment may be

verbal or through your thoughts at this time but remain in your seated, restful position with little movement, if any.

6. Observe the animal quietly. Notice body language, expressions, and overall demeanor as you continue to breathe lightly, continuing to focus energy into your own central core.

7. When the animal's demeanor is calm, relaxed, trusting, approaching, or inquisitive (or a combination of these), introduce yourself and express your desire to communicate with them. You may do so verbally or through telepathy.

- Telepathy is simply a means of non-verbal communication using images, energy, or sensations you believe the animal will understand. "Ball," for example, is an image many dogs connect with not only a specific toy but also the act of play. Using telepathic communication works best when images, energy, or sensations are directed from your mind (specifically in between your eyes) to the mind of the animal (specifically in between their eyes). Keep in mind that animals are the most fluent in images.

- If, however, you have a name for the object and act as well as a visual, this is the best way to start learning the animal's specific language. For example: ball=red tennis ball=Elmo Ball=park ball. When this specific dog hears, visualizes, or touches "ball," he infers everything else connected with it. A different dog might have a completely different, even negative reaction, to the same word or image.

- Working with an animal you know well, then, is the best way to get started with learning the art of animal communication. Once you have mastered the nature of the language, you will quickly be able to adapt to different dialects.

8. Be receptive to any images, sensations, emotions, or words you may receive. It takes time to filter genuine responses from the ones created in our minds, particularly if there is no way to confirm information, but practice and patience will hone your skills. You will be able to "think" to your animal companion and they will have a tangible, physical response!

9. Pull back your energetic connection gently as you thank the animal for the sacred time you have spent together.
10. Take several deep breaths in through your nose and out through your mouth, reconnecting to the physical space around you, grounding your physical form, and rebalancing your energy as you allow the energy you have built up to dissipate.
11. Provide reassurance, support, and understanding based on the insights you have gained from the session. Just as with any communication, if a desire or concern is expressed and no action is taken, further attempts at communication may be less successful.

Once you have mastered the art of communication with your own pet, you may begin working with other animals following the same guidelines. Keep in mind that you will need to learn the basics of their language as well as establish trust in order to begin a fruitful process.

Patience and practice will help you strengthen your filters and build the arsenal of tools you will need to become an excellent animal communicator.

5 HEALING SPACE

Creating a sacred space for Reiki work is a foundational step in facilitating healing and energy flow. This space serves as a vessel for the transformative energies of Reiki, allowing them to flow freely and with intention. In this chapter, we will explore the essential elements and steps to craft a nurturing environment conducive to a productive and healing session.

Selecting the right location is crucial in establishing a sacred healing space for Reiki work. Consider the following factors:

- Quiet & Peaceful: Choose an area free from disturbances and noise, where both practitioner and recipient can relax without disruptions. Turn off cell phones and disconnect doorbells or put on silent as possible.
- Well-Ventilated & Comfortable: Ensure the space has good airflow and temperature control to create a comfortable environment for both the practitioner and recipient.
- Natural or Soft Lighting: If possible, choose a space with access to natural light.

Before infusing the space with Reiki energy, it is important to clear any residual or stagnant energies. It is important to do so prior to beginning the process of connecting with and anchoring Reiki's light. This can be achieved through various methods:

- Smudging: Open a window or door and light a smudging stick such as White Sage or Palo Santo and allow the smoke to cleanse the space as it burns, move clockwise in a spiral, starting in the center of the space and spreading outward, paying special attention to corners and other less-used areas of the space.

- Holy Water: Using Holy Water and sacred prayers, move clockwise in the space, starting at the threshold of the room and ending in the same location. Be sure to mist the walls, ceiling, and floor along the way as you speak your prayers aloud.

- If the session is performed outside, creating a perimeter with four clear quartz crystal points will keep the energy you build in your sacred space. Choose a location that feels energetically sound. Place your first crystal and place it, point up, at the north as you say a sacred prayer. Continue your prayer as you continue clockwise around your circle, placing a crystal the same way in each quadrant and completing your prayer at the north.

If you will be using music or aromatherapy for your session, it is important to make careful selections and utilize them sparingly. Remember that some essential oils are toxic to animals, and certain sounds or music may be distracting.

Every client will be different, so you will need to use your intuition to guide you in this process. When I work with my animal clients, I rarely choose to use music or aromatherapy in active sessions. I will often recommend certain essential oils or even tumbled stones for post-session use, however, dependent upon the issues I encounter.

At the conclusion of a session, it is important to close the healing space. Gently disconnect from the energy and the space itself with an attitude of gratitude and grace. Visualize the location bathed in a radiant and protective light, ensuring it remains a sacred and nurturing environment for as long as it can naturally be sustained.

This spot may be used again for subsequent sessions, but do plan to prepare it as before, to clear out any unwanted energy that may have accumulated during your time away.

Your animal (or human) client will be drawn to this space, as it is now a hub of positive and healing light which will continue to gently supplement the session you have performed.

A sacred healing space is the canvas upon which Reiki energy unfolds its transformative potential. By attending to every detail, from the physical elements to the energetic intention, practitioners create an environment that supports deep healing and rejuvenation for both them and their clients. The nurturing space becomes a sanctuary for the profound work of Reiki.

6 A PRACTITIONER'S ROLE

At the heart of Reiki practice lies the profound role of the practitioner as a conduit for Universal Life Force Energy. This energy, the very essence of life itself, flows through the practitioner, facilitating healing, balance, and transformation. It is a sacred responsibility and privilege.

As a Reiki practitioner, one assumes the sacred duty of holding a space of love, compassion, and non-judgment. This allows the recipient to release, heal, and grow, knowing they are fully supported by the promise of restoration and harmonization.

Being present is a cornerstone of the practitioner's sacred role. By fully immersing themselves in the here and now, practitioners create a space where time fades, and healing becomes a timeless dance between energy and intention.

The practitioner respects and honors the unique journey of each recipient. They understand that healing is a deeply personal process, and they approach it with humility, allowing the recipient's innate wisdom to guide the way. Those who practice healing arts know that they cannot heal anyone. They are simply the mediators of energy, opening doorways and facilitating the transmission of correct rays.

The recipient must desire and receive the energy and then accept it, *use* it for the healing process.

The role of the practitioner extends beyond the session itself. It encompasses empowering the recipient to take an active role in their own healing journey. Practitioners share tools, insights, and guidance that enable recipients to continue their path of self-discovery and healing.

When the client is an animal, all this information can be communicated to the animal and his/her human, so that appropriate steps can be taken for full participation in the healing process.

The sacred practitioner acknowledges and respects the autonomy of the recipient. They offer Reiki with an open heart, without attachment to specific outcomes.

To be in service is also to recognize the importance of personal growth and self-care. Practitioners must tend to their own well-being, ensuring they remain vessels of harmonious energy for the benefit of all living things.

Every session, every interaction, and every moment as a Reiki practitioner is an opportunity for gratitude and healing. Practitioners cultivate reverence for the gift they share and facilitate.

The sacred role is a profound calling, a path of service, and a journey of deep spiritual growth. It is both a privilege and a responsibility to walk this path of reverence as an instrument of Light.

7 SACRED ENERGY

I have been privileged to practice various forms of Reiki across the United States as well as in various countries over the past 20 years. As a practitioner, I have seen some wondrous things occur with both animal and human clients, as well as being honored with some beautiful communications.

But each session, each client, is sacred and new. Each provides me with an opportunity to grow as a practitioner, to learn, to heal, and to represent the work I cherish so much with passion and heart.

There have been times I doubted my connection, my ability to anchor the sacred ray. But each of these moments, as I breathed and trusted, was followed by a shift in the client that was palpable.

It took me years to fully understand that it was my own resistance to the Light, my judgment of myself, and my skills, that was stopping the flow of Reiki in those moments.

Reiki must flow without expectation of result. The moment the practitioner pushes…energy stops. This is the nature of "ki" and the vibration of healing versus the lack of vibration made by blockages.

In the practice of Reiki, blockages are not removed by force, doubt, or mere intention. They cannot be torn out or blasted away. They are to be addressed with the purest, most precious ray of Light and delicately dissolved, carefully absorbed, and balanced, harmonized, and stabilized.

The practitioner is trained to identify blockages and also in the surgical direction of the ray. But only by understanding the nature of energy and how to work with it as it courses through different planes, can the practitioner truly master this ancient art.

The infusion of Reiki Light opens the gateways for deep, lasting healing on the physical, emotional, mental, and spiritual levels. And one does not need to be a master to experience its beauty or healing power.

Novice practitioners, particularly children, have demonstrated themselves to be quite adept at this art. Perhaps it is their willingness to let go of expectations? Perhaps it is the purity of their channels? Perhaps it is their connection to their intuitiveness? Perhaps a combination of all three.

Regardless, it is something to note. Those of us on the Reiki path are life-long students. We are seekers of divine knowledge and bringers of harmony and balance.

Reiki is more than a path of healing. It is a path of hope.

ABOUT THE AUTHOR

Elizabeth Selden is a teacher, guest speaker, podcaster, post-trauma empowerment specialist, and alternative health practitioner with over thirty years of experience in the study, exploration, and integration of ancient holistic therapies and their origins.

She works with animals and their humans alike to support the healing of the "whole being," with Reiki as a foundational building block for other therapies.

www.ingramcontent.com/pod-product-compliance
Lightning Source LLC
Chambersburg PA
CBHW070756260726
48660CB00007B/3154